USMLE STEP 2 CK
Pediatrics
In Your Pocket

✓ Study guide for the USMLE STEP 2 CK exam.
✓ Prepare for your shelf examination.
✓ Be ready for your inpatient rotation.

Gregory J. Fernandez M.D.

First Edition, 2016

Author & Editor: Gregory J. Fernandez, M.D.

Publisher: M.D. Educational Services

Peer-review: Sumayya Aboobacker, MBBS ,FICM. College of Clinical Medicine, China, Three Gorges University & Dr. Kamleshun Ramphul, M.D Pediatrics, Shanghai Jiao Tong University School of Medicine.

Book Design: Marie Meyer and Di Freeze

Copyediting: Editage Cactus Communications

DISCLAIMER: The author, editor, publisher, and staff members have taken care to confirm the accuracy of the information present in this publication. The context of the books entirety, is believed to be reliable in accordance with the standards accepted at the time of publication. However, readers are encouraged to confirm the information and conduct their own research for clarification of all the information present within this book. No one involved in creating this book is responsible for errors or omissions or for any consequences from application of the information in this book. There is no warranty, expressed or implied, with respect to the completeness or accuracy of the contents of this publication. Neither the editor, nor the author assumes any liability for any injury and/or damage to persons or property arising from the content of this publication. Application of this information in a particular situation remains the professional responsibility of the practitioner; the clinical treatments or information described and recommended may not be considered absolute and universal recommendations. It is the responsibility of the health care provider to ascertain the FDA status of each drug used or device planned for use in their clinical practice. The purpose of this books, is to be used as a study guide for medical examinations. Please consult with attending physicians for any medical decisions.

ISBN-13: 978-1530479221

ISBN-10: 1530479223

This book is gratefully dedicated to my wife. Thank you for your support and always being there for me. Thank you for your kindness, your devotion, and your endless selflessness support. I love you... Thank you mother, father, step-mother, brothers, friends, and family for all your encouragement and endless love. Best of luck to all the medical dreamers, the road is long and I hope my book helps you through this journey. All the best...

How to Use
"Pediatrics In Your Pocket"

Pediatrics in Your Pocket is a study guide for the USMLE STEP 2 CK exam that you can also use to prepare for your shelf examination and to get ready for your inpatient rotation. It is part of a series, each dealing with a different subject or sub-specialty, focusing on vital clinical knowledge.

The subjects and topics within pediatrics are called out in large, colored type. These items are also included in the Table of Contents for ease of access.

Many subjects also contain sub-subjects that are called out in bold, blue

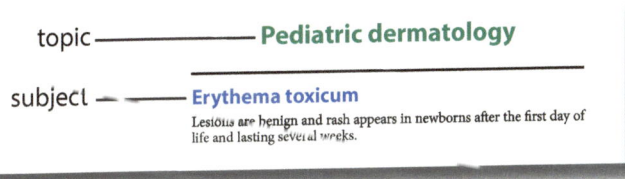

topic ——————— **Pediatric dermatology**

subject — —— **Erythema toxicum**
Lesions are benign and rash appears in newborns after the first day of life and lasting several weeks.

type, either as bulleted items or in-line with the text, as appropriate. They are all referenced in the index.

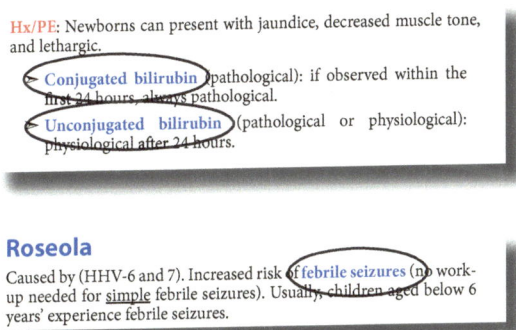

Hx/PE: Newborns can present with jaundice, decreased muscle tone, and lethargic.
- **Conjugated bilirubin** (pathological): if observed within the first 24 hours, always pathological.
- **Unconjugated bilirubin** (pathological or physiological): physiological after 24 hours.

Roseola
Caused by (HHV-6 and 7). Increased risk of febrile seizures (no work-up needed for simple febrile seizures). Usually, children aged below 6 years' experience febrile seizures.

Presentation of clinical history and physical exam (Hx/PE), step-by-step diagnosis, and treatment plan are indicated by bold red headings.

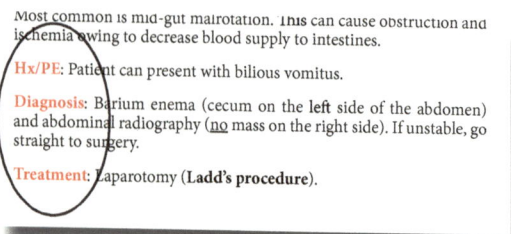

Most common is mid-gut malrotation. This can cause obstruction and ischemia owing to decrease blood supply to intestines.

Hx/PE: Patient can present with bilious vomitus.

Diagnosis: Barium enema (cecum on the left side of the abdomen) and abdominal radiography (no mass on the right side). If unstable, go straight to surgery.

Treatment: Laparotomy (**Ladd's procedure**).

Procedures, triads, pathology, medications, antibodies and findings are called out in bold text. These items are also included in the index.

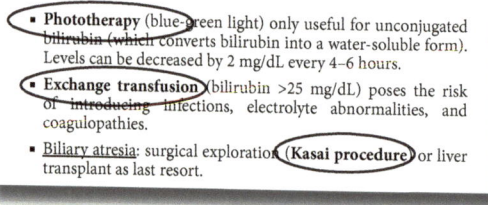

- **Phototherapy** (blue-green light) only useful for unconjugated bilirubin (which converts bilirubin into a water-soluble form). Levels can be decreased by 2 mg/dL every 4–6 hours.
- **Exchange transfusion** (bilirubin >25 mg/dL) poses the risk of introducing infections, electrolyte abnormalities, and coagulopathies.
- Biliary atresia: surgical exploration (**Kasai procedure**) or liver transplant as last resort.

Reflexes, signs and maneuvers are shown in purple text.

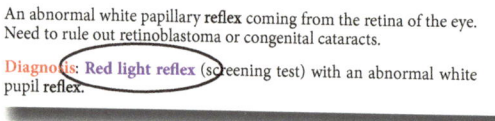

An abnormal white papillary **reflex** coming from the retina of the eye. Need to rule out retinoblastoma or congenital cataracts.

Diagnosis: **Red light reflex** (screening test) with an abnormal white pupil **reflex**.

Mnemonics and key words are shown in orange text.

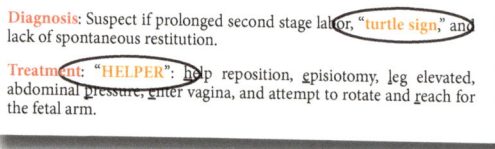

Diagnosis: Suspect if prolonged second stage labor, "turtle sign," and lack of spontaneous restitution.

Treatment: "HELPER": help reposition, episiotomy, leg elevated, abdominal pressure, enter vagina, and attempt to rotate and reach for the fetal arm.

And, finally, for the avoidance of doubt, circumstances that amount to a medical emergency are flagged with a warning.

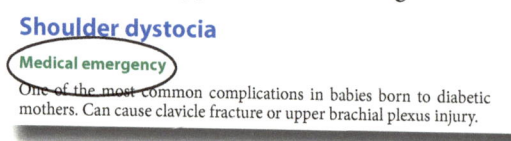

Shoulder dystocia

Medical emergency

One of the most common complications in babies born to diabetic mothers. Can cause clavicle fracture or upper brachial plexus injury.

Pediatrics
Table of Contents

Neonates 1
Normal vital signs 1
APGAR score............................ 1
Management at delivery 2
Transient tachypnea of newborn
(TTN) 2
Infant respiratory distress syndrome
(RDS) 2
Jaundice 3
Bile acids of newborn 4
Vitamin K deficiency 4
Vitamin D................................ 5
Hepatitis B vaccination............... 5
Conjunctivitis 5
Screening for newborns 6
Developing reflexes...................... 7

Injuries to newborns 7
Subconjunctival hemorrhage......... 7
Skull fractures 7
Caput succedaneum..................... 8
Erb-Duchenne palsy 8
Klumpke's palsy 8
Clavicular fracture 9
Shoulder dystocia........................ 9

Pediatric dermatology.................. 9
Erythema toxicum 9
Mongolian spots......................... 10
Diaper dermatitis 10
Diaper candidiasis...................... 10

Pediatric cardiology 11
Ventricular septal defect (VSD) ... 11
Atrial septal defect (ASD) 12
Patent ductus arteriosus (PDA).... 12
Coarctation of aorta..................... 13
Transposition of the great arteries 14
Tetralogy of Fallot (ToF) 15
Total anomalous pulmonary venous
return (TAPVR) 15
Truncus arteriosus 16
Tricuspid atresia 16
Third heart sounds...................... 17
Children with systolic murmurs .. 17

Renovascular disease 17

Genetic defects............................ 17
Down syndrome........................... 17
Edwards syndrome 18
Patau syndrome........................... 19
Klinefelter syndrome 20
Turner syndrome.......................... 20
Phenylketonuria (PKU) 21
McCune-Albright syndrome 21
Fragile X syndrome...................... 22
Cystic fibrosis (CF) 22

Pediatric gastroenterology 23
Choanal atresia........................... 23
Tracheal esophageal fistula 23
Congenital diaphragmatic hernia 24
Gastroschisis.............................. 25
Omphalocele............................... 25
Pyloric stenosis........................... 26
Duodenal atresia 26
Volvulus..................................... 27
Intussusception........................... 27
Malrotation 28
Meckel's diverticulum.................. 29
Hirschsprung's disease................. 29
Necrotizing enterocolitis (NEC) .. 30
Congenital umbilical hernias 30
Gastroesophageal reflux in child.. 31
Constipation in children 31
Acute diarrhea in children........... 32
Obesity in children 32

Pediatric immunological disorders
....32
Bruton's agammaglobulinemia..... 32
Common variable immunodefi-
ciency...................................... 33
IgA deficiency............................. 33
Wiskott-Aldrich syndrome.......... 33
Chronic granulomatous disease
(CGD)...................................... 34
DiGeorge syndrome..................... 34

cont'd on next page

Pediatrics
Table of Contents, cont'd

Ataxia-telangiectasia 35
Severe combined immunodeficiency (SCID) 35
Leukocyte adhesion deficiency (LAD) 35
Chediak–Higashi syndrome 36
C1 esterase deficiency 36
Terminal complement deficiency 36

Pediatric infectious diseases 37
Bronchiolitis 37
Croup (laryngotracheobronchitis) 38
Epiglottitis 39
Retropharyngeal abscess 39
Pertussis (whooping cough) 39
Meningitis in children 40
Urinary tract infection in children 41
Erythema infectiosum (parvovirus B19) 42
Measles 43
Mumps.. 43
Rubella.. 43
Roseola 44
Varicella...................................... 44
Zoster.. 45
Hand-foot-mouth disease 46
Kawasaki disease 46
Cerebral palsy 47

Pediatric fever........................... 47
Febrile seizures 47

Pediatric cancers....................... 48
Leukemia.................................... 48
Neuroblastoma 49
Wilms' tumor.............................. 49
Ewing's sarcoma 50
Osteosarcoma 50
Von Hippel-Lindau syndrome (VHL)...................................... 51
Sarcoma botryoides 51

Pediatric nutrition deficiency ... 51
Rickets 51
Common vitamin deficiencies in children....................................... 52

Pediatric genetic disease........... 53
Vitamin D-dependent rickets (type I)...................................... 53
Prader-Willi syndrome............... 53
Friedreich's ataxia...................... 53
Henoch-Schonlein purpura........ 54
Sudden infant death syndrome .. 54

Pediatric ophthalmology........... 54
Amblyopia................................... 54
Strabismus.................................. 55
Leukocoria 55
Retinoblastoma (RB) 55
Dacryostenosis 56

Pediatric poisoning 56
Reye's syndrome 56
Lead poisoning 57

Pediatric congenital disorders .. 57
Thymic shadow........................... 57
Nasal polyps................................ 58
Thyroglossal duct cyst 58
Brachial cleft cyst 58
Cystic hygroma........................... 59

Pediatric enuresis 59
Primary enuresis 59
Secondary enuresis 59

Pediatric development.............. 60
Milestones 60

Pediatric vaccinations 61
Vaccinations............................... 61

Childhood injury prevention.... 62
Preventative measures 62

Neonates

Normal vital signs

➤ Normal newborn respiratory rate: 30–50 respirations per minute.

➤ Normal newborn heart rate: 100–160 beats per minute.

➤ Normal blood pressure (age 1-12 months): systolic 75-100 mmHg and diastolic 50-70 mmHg.

➤ Oral temperature: 98.0° F - 98.6° F and 1° F higher for rectal measurement.

APGAR score

Measure APGAR at 1 minute and 5 minutes or continued intervals if needed. Total possible points 10.

Points:

➤ 7 10 (good health).

➤ 4–6 (stimulate and observation).

➤ 0–3 (resuscitation).

Category	0 points	1 point	2 points
Appearance (color)	Blue all over.	Pink in trunk.	Pink all over.
Pulse (rate)	Asystole.	<100 bpm.	>100 bpm.
Grimace (reflex)	No response.	Mild grimace.	Cough/strong grimace
Activity (muscle tone)	None.	Some flexion.	Active movements.
Respiration (breathing)	Absent	Irregular or weak pulse.	Regular.

Management at delivery

➤ 0.5% erythromycin ophthalmic ointment (prevents bacterial conjunctivitis).

➤ 1 mg of IM vitamin K (prevents hemorrhage).

➤ Hepatitis B vaccine to neonate, if mother is hepatitis B-negative.

  • <u>Add</u> hepatitis IVIG (within 12 hours) if mother is HBsAg-positive.

Transient tachypnea of newborn (TTN)

Respiratory distress caused by delayed reabsorption of fetal lung fluid. Common if rapid second stage of labor, prematurity, or C-section. Usually resolves within 12–24 hours but can last up to 72 hours in severe cases.

Hx/PE: Tachypnea, tachycardia, nasal flaring, and costal retractions.

Diagnosis: If tachypnea lasts >4 hours consider a full septic work-up: CBC, electrolytes, pulse oximetry, ABG, blood culture, urinalysis, urine culture, lumbar puncture (rare, unless high suspicion or display of neurological signs), and chest radiography.

Treatment: Usually supportive measures (such as oxygen) and close observation.

Infant respiratory distress syndrome (RDS)

More common in neonates born between 28–34 weeks, as during this stage they have decreased surfactant levels that leads to decreased lung compliance and atelectasis. Surfactant (*type II pneumocytes*) decreases surface tension and prevents alveoli collapse.

Hx/PE: Respiratory rate >60 per/min (respiratory alkalosis), nasal flaring, and intercostal retractions.

Diagnosis:

  ▪ CBC, ABG (respiratory alkalosis), and blood culture.

  ▪ *Best initial test*: chest radiography ("**ground glass**" appearance).

  ▪ *Best predictive test*: **lecithin-sphingomyelin ratio** (L/S ratio).

Treatment:

- *Best initial therapy*: oxygen and possible nasal CPAP or intubation.
- *Most effective treatment*: artificial exogenous surfactant (*decreases mortality*).
- If premature, give mother dexamethasone IM (preferably 2 doses within 24 hours prior to delivery).
  - <34 weeks (IM steroids to mother and consider tocolytics).
  - >34 weeks (L/S ratio to determine lung maturity).

Note:

✓ TTN → fetal lung fluid/amniotic fluid).

✓ Meconium aspiration → meconium aspiration in utero.

✓ RDS → low surfactant.

Jaundice

Can be caused by increased hemolysis, increased production of bilirubin, or decreased excretion of bilirubin.

Types:

➤ Conjugated bilirubin (pathological): if observed within the first 24 hours, always pathological.

➤ Unconjugated bilirubin (pathological or physiological): physiological after 24 hours.

Kernicterus: unconjugated (indirect) bilirubin accumulation in pons or basal ganglion, which can present with high-pitch cry, hypotonia, and seizures.

Hx/PE: Newborns can present with jaundice, decreased muscle tone, and lethargic.

Diagnosis:

- CBC with blood smears, direct and total bilirubin levels, blood type of mother and infant (ABO and Rh incompatibility), and Coomb's test.
- Biliary atresia: elevated LFTs and **phenobarbital-enhanced hepatobiliary scintigraphy**.

Note: Rh incompatibility is more severe than ABO incompatibility.

Treatment:

- **Phototherapy** (blue-green light) only useful for unconjugated bilirubin (which converts bilirubin into a water-soluble form). Levels can be decreased by 2 mg/dL every 4–6 hours.

- **Exchange transfusion** (bilirubin >25 mg/dL) poses the risk of introducing infections, electrolyte abnormalities, and coagulopathies.

- Biliary atresia: surgical exploration (**Kasai procedure**) or liver transplant as last resort.

Note:

➤ Physiological jaundice: occurs after 24 hours of birth.

➤ Biliary atresia (elevated LFTs) and erythroblastosis fetalis: (occur within the first 24 hours of birth).

➤ Breastfeeding jaundice: caused by inadequate feeding = dehydration = dry appearing baby.

➤ Milk-induced jaundice: usually takes at least a week. Mothers are encouraged to continue the feeding regiment, since this jaundice is self-limiting. No need for breastfeeding cessation. However, some studies recommend stopping breastfeeding for a few days with formula supplementation and restart breastfeeding later.

Bile acids of newborn

Bile acid content is less in neonates and may present with steatorrhea, watery stools, and decreased weight gain. This is one of the reasons why babies have diarrhea and weight loss in the first few days of life.

Vitamin K deficiency

The gut of neonates is not adequately colonized by *E. coli*; therefore, they do not have sufficient quantities of vitamin K.

Diagnosis: Increased bleeding after umbilical cord is cut or after circumcision.

Treatment: Routine administration of 1mg of vitamin K (IM) is given shortly after birth to avoid hemorrhagic disease.

Note: Need consent from mother for vitamin K injection.

Vitamin D

Breast milk in humans is low in vitamin D.

Treatment: All babies who are breastfeeding need supplementation of vitamin D (400 IU/mL) <u>or</u> fortified formula added to their diet with a similar dosage.

Hepatitis B vaccination

➤ Every child should get a hepatitis B vaccination before discharge, at 2 months, and again at 6 months of age. A mother can refuse vaccinations and should be documented in the patient chart.

➤ If the mother tests <u>positive</u> for hepatitis B, the newborn should get the vaccination <u>plus</u> an additional hepatitis B immunoglobulin (within 12 hours). Re-test for hepatitis B serology at 9-15 months of age.

Conjunctivitis

Conjunctivitis time-line:

➤ Conjunctivitis on the first day of life is most likely caused by chemical irritation (example prophylactic eye drops).

➤ 2–7 days – most likely *Neisseria gonorrhoeae*.

➤ >7 days – most likely *Chlamydia trachomatis* ("neovascularization" on physical examination).

➤ 3 weeks – most likely herpes virus ("dendritic ulcers" on physical examination).

Diagnosis: Conjunctival scraping with use of Gram stain and PCR.

Treatment:
- Chemical conjunctivitis: not usually treated.
- *N gonorrhoeae conjunctivitis:* use cephalosporins.
- *C. trachomatis* conjunctivitis: give <u>oral</u> erythromycin, which also decreases the risk of chlamydial pneumonia. History

of chlamydia conjunctivitis is extremely important in the diagnosis of chlamydia pneumonia.

Note:

✓ Chlamydia pneumonia is also treated with <u>oral</u> erythromycin.

✓ Do not give doxycycline to children younger than 8 years of age.

✓ Silver nitrate solution can cause chemical conjunctivitis.

<u>Prevention</u>: At birth, give 0.5% erythromycin drops (commonly used) or silver nitrate solution (not as commonly used).

Screening for newborns

Newborn screening varies from one state to another.

"**Please check before going home**": <u>P</u>KU, <u>c</u>ongenital adrenal hyperplasia, <u>b</u>iotin deficiency, galactosemia, and <u>h</u>omocystinuria/<u>h</u>ypothyroidism. Need to also conduct a hearing test and red light reflex.

Note: Hearing test should be performed at birth (controversial); visual testing to be done before 6 years of age but recommended at least by 3 years. Red light reflex needs to be done before discharge.

Diagnosis: Screen newborn for genetic abnormalities (blood sample), hearing loss (hearing test), Retinoblastoma (red light reflex), and congenital heart disease (pulse oximetry).

Treatment:
- <u>PKU</u>: low phenylalanine diet and increased tyrosine in diet.
- <u>Congenital adrenal hyperplasia</u>: mineralocorticoids plus glucocorticoids and genital reconstruction, if needed. Treatment depends on type of adrenal hyperplasia.
- <u>Hypothyroidism</u>: levothyroxine.
- <u>Galactosemia</u>: decrease lactose-containing products (do not breastfeed).
- <u>Hearing test</u>: should be done within the first month.
- <u>Pulse oximetry</u>: used to rule out congenital heart disease.

Developing reflexes

- **Moro reflex**: when baby is startled, they spread their arms symmetrically.
- **Rotting reflex**: when cheek is touched, baby should turn to that side.
- **Sucking reflex**: baby automatically sucks on nipple-shaped objects.
- **Babinski reflex**: toe extension upwards (normal only in babies and abnormal in adults).
- **Superman reflex**: when held facing the floor, arms move outwards.
- **Grasping reflex**: when an object is placed in palm, they will grasp object.

Injuries to newborns

Subconjunctival hemorrhage

Ocular trauma caused by labor compressions.

Hx/PE: Sharply marked bright red area over the sclera.

Diagnosis: Clinical diagnosis.

Treatment: Observation.

Skull fractures

Types:

- Linear (most common).
- Depressed.
- Basilar (most fatal).

Caput succedaneum

Soft tissue swelling of the scalp that <u>does</u> cross the suture lines.

Diagnosis: Clinical diagnosis.

Treatment: Improves within weeks to months.

Erb-Duchenne palsy

Nerve involvement of the <u>upper</u> trunk of the brachial plexus (C5-C6) caused by forceful stretching of the head and shoulder. Can cause damage to the <u>phrenic nerve</u> causing diaphragmatic paralysis (cranial nerves C3- C5).

Hx/PE: Arm is pronated and medially rotated. "Waiter's tip" posture.

Diagnosis: Clinical diagnosis.

Treatment:

- Immobilization followed by physical therapy is the *best treatment.*
- If no improvement in 3-6 months then consider nerve surgery.
- Monitor respiration.

Note: Prognosis is good with an 80% recovery rate. Only a few will develop complications.

Klumpke's palsy

Nerve involvement of the <u>lower</u> trunk of the brachial plexus (C8-T1), caused from sudden upward pulling of the arm resulting in nerve damage. The <u>median</u> and <u>ulnar</u> nerves are primarily the nerves damaged which mainly effect the muscles of the hands. "Claw hand" posture.

Hx/PE: T1 involvement may result in Horner's syndrome.

Diagnosis: Clinical diagnosis.

Treatment:
- Immobilization followed by physical therapy is the *best treatment*.
- If no improvement in 3-6 months consider surgery.

Clavicular fracture

Most common newborn fracture and commonly caused by shoulder dystocia. May cause injury to brachial plexus.

Diagnosis: Baby gram or ultrasound image.

Treatment: Immobilization and physical therapy.

Shoulder dystocia

Medical emergency

One of the most common complications in babies born to diabetic mothers. Can cause clavicle fracture or brachial plexus injury.

Risks factors: Babies born to diabetic mothers, obesity in mothers, male fetus, and macrosomia.

Diagnosis: Suspect if prolonged second stage of labor, "turtle sign," and lack of spontaneous restitution.

Treatment: "HELPER": help reposition, episiotomy, leg elevated, abdominal pressure, enter vagina, and attempt to rotate and reach for the fetal arm.

Zavanelli's maneuver → placing baby back in the uterus, followed by performing a cesarean section).

Pediatric dermatology

Erythema toxicum

Lesions are benign and rash appears in newborns during the first days of life and lasting several weeks.

Hx/PE: Erythematous base with white papules (which are full of eosinophils).

Diagnosis: Clinical diagnosis or scraping of lesion.

Treatment: Self-limited.

Mongolian spots

<u>Benign</u> congenital birth mark more common in Koreans.

Hx/PE: Flat blue/gray macules more commonly located on the presacral region.

Diagnosis: Clinical diagnosis. Need to rule out child abuse if high suspicion.

Treatment: No treatment and usually vanishes by the age of 3 years.

Diaper dermatitis

Usually caused by contact dermatitis from fecal and urinary irritation.

Hx/PE: Usually does <u>not</u> involve the skin folds.

Diagnosis: Clinical diagnosis or KOH culture, if unsure.

Treatment:

- Bathing with mild soaps and water and frequent diaper changes. Remove diaper to allow skin to dry.
- May require petroleum ointment, low-strength corticosteroids, or topical zinc oxide paste.

Diaper candidiasis

Demarcated papules and plaques in the diaper area, rather than shiny areas of erythema seen in dermatitis. Usually involves the skin folds.

Diagnosis: Clinical diagnosis or KOH culture (if needed to confirm diagnosis).

Treatment: Topical antifungal (**clotrimazole cream**).

Pediatric cardiology

Ventricular septal defect (VSD)

Incomplete formation of the *interventricular septum* creating a holosystolic murmur. At first, presents as a left to right shunt (best heard in the right lower sternal border) and then followed by a right to left shunt (best heard in the left lower sternal border). This is the *most common* congenital cardiac defect and is common in trisomy's disease.

Hx/PE: Murmur increases with squatting, hand gripping, and leg elevation. Can present with increased respiratory infection, SOB, FTT, and CHF.

Note:

✓ If a large shunt, can have a softer sounding murmur.

✓ If a smaller shunt, can have a louder sounding murmur.

Diagnosis:

- EKG: first develops right ventricular hypertrophy (RVH) followed by left ventricular hypertrophy (LVH) as disease progresses.

  - Hypertrophy will depend on where the fluids are going.

- Chest radiography: increased pulmonary vascular markings (later stages).

- Echocardiogram (*gold standard*, *most useful*, and *best initial test*): left to right shunt, which progresses to a right to left shunt.

- **Cardiac catheterization** is *more accurate* than echocardiogram but more invasive and not as commonly used.

Treatment:

- About 50% close spontaneously within the first 6 months (need echocardiogram monitoring).

- Diuretics, ACEi, and digoxin can be helpful if symptomatic.

- Surgery required if progresses to development of pulmonary hypertension, CHF, or long standing defect.

Atrial septal defect (ASD)

Most common type is patent foramen ovale, which carries risk of paradoxical embolus. Causes a left sternal systolic murmur best heard in the left upper sternal border.

Risk of developing arrhythmias, SOB, FTT, CHF, pulmonary hypertension, and increased frequency of respiratory infections.

Types:
- ➤ **Ostium primary defect** (less common).
- ➤ **Ostium secondary defect** (more common).

Hx/PE: "**Fixed wide splitting of S2**," large defects (>9mm) are more difficult to hear on physical examination.

Diagnosis:
- EKG: first right axis deviation, which can later become left axis. Can present with arrhythmias.
- Chest radiography: increased pulmonary vascular markings (later stages).
- Echocardiogram (*gold standard* and *best initial test*): left to right shunt, which later develops into a right to left shunt.

Treatment:
- Majority close spontaneously.
- If smaller than 8 mm, can be monitored in the first 2 years of life.
- Diuretics can be helpful to decrease fluid load and work load on heart.
- Might consider antiplatelet medications to prevent coagulations.
- Surgery required if patient develops CHF (2:1 pulmonary to systemic ratio) or pulmonary hypertension.

Patent ductus arteriosus (PDA)

A congenital heart disease where the ductus arteriosus fails to close. Blood flows between the *aorta* and *pulmonary artery*. More common in females and can be associated with rubella infections.

Hx/PE: Load S2 with a systolic murmur that spills into a diastolic murmur causing a "machine-like" murmur creating wide and bounding pulses.

Diagnosis:

- EKG: left ventricular axis.

- Chest radiography: cardiomegaly.

- Echocardiogram: left ventricle and left atrial enlargement (most useful).

- Doppler studies: blood flows between the aorta and pulmonary artery (*gold standard*).

Note: PDA can be a normal finding in the first 12 hours of life (especially in premature infants) but after 24 hours of life needs to be investigated, if does not close spontaneously.

Treatment:

- If caused by premature birth, administer indomethacin ([NSAIDs] <u>inhibits</u> prostaglandins, useful medication to close duct).

- Prostaglandins can keep the PDA open when needed.

- If indomethacin fails or >6–8 months, surgical correction is needed with ductal ligation.

Coarctation of aorta

A congenital disease where the aorta narrows near the ductus arteriosus and can be associated with Turner syndrome (5%) and Berry aneurysms.

<u>Types</u>:

➤ <u>Preductal</u> (children): proximal narrowing from the ductus arteriosus.

➤ <u>Postductal</u> (adults): distal narrowing from the ductus arteriosus. Associated with rib notching.

Hx/PE: Decreased lower extremity pulses with exacerbation of upper extremity pulses and blood pressure differences between both upper extremities. Systolic murmur loudest below the left scapula and radiates to the left axilla.

Diagnosis:

- EKG: left axis.
- Chest radiography: pulmonary congestion, cardiomegaly, and posterior rib notching (postductal).
- Doppler studies and echocardiogram (*gold standard*).

Treatment:

- Keep PDA open with PGE1 (to help ensure lower extremity blood flow).
- Surgical repair (after stabilization) or balloon angioplasty (controversial).
- Monitor for brain aneurysm, cardiac tamponade, and aortic dissection.

Transposition of the great arteries

The aorta arises from the right ventricle and the pulmonary artery from the left ventricle. Common in diabetic mothers. The exchange of oxygenated blood is via the PDA, ASD, and/or VSD.

Hx/PE: Patient presents with shortness of breath soon after birth with a single S2 heart sound.

Diagnosis:

- Chest radiography: straight or narrow mediastinum with increased pulmonary blood flow. "Egg on a string appearance."
- Echocardiogram (*gold standard*).
- Cardiac catheterization is usually ordered when additional information is needed.

Treatment:

- IV PGE1 to keep PDA open.
- **Balloon atrial septostomy** (opens foramen ovale) allows mixture of oxygenated and deoxygenated blood.
- If VSD is present, leave open.

Note: Part of the emergency management is intravenous infusion of prostaglandin E1 to keep the PDA open. NSAIDs are contraindicated because will cause closure of the ductus.

Tetralogy of Fallot (ToF)

A congenital heart disease and commonly associated with chromosome 22 disorders. Involves common tetrad: "PROV" pulmonary stenosis, RVH, over-riding aorta, and VSD.

Hx/PE: Tet-spells (hypercyanotic spells, self-limited, lasting fewer than 10–15 minutes) which are characterized by sudden cyanosis secondary to decrease systemic vascular resistance, which causes increase venous return and leads to increase shunting of blood.

Diagnosis:
- EKG: right ventricular hypertrophy and right axis deviation.
- Chest radiography: "boot shaped heart" and decreased pulmonary markings.
- Echocardiogram (*gold standard*).

Treatment:
- Oxygen, morphine sulfate, and knee-chest position (increases systemic vascular resistance).
- Tet spells can be treated with epinephrine or norepinephrine to increase systemic resistances.
- Surgical intervention (usually between 4 and 12 months) is the only *definitive therapy.*

Total anomalous pulmonary venous return (TAPVR)

Pulmonary veins forming a confluence behind the left atrium and draining into the right atrium. Causes a mixture of deoxygenated and oxygenated blood.

Hx/PE: Mild cyanosis initially then later presents with CHF and arrhythmias.

Diagnosis:
- EKG: right axis deviation and possible arrhythmias.
- Chest radiography: increased pulmonary markings (actually very difficult to see on x-ray).

- Echocardiogram: right atrial enlargement.

Treatment: Give PGE1 (keep ductus arteriosus open) and surgery is *definitive* (can be done within the first month after birth).

Truncus arteriosus

Truncus arteriosus when a <u>single</u> trunk emerges from both right and left ventricles and gives rise to all major circulation.

Hx/PE: Symptoms appear within the first few days of life with dyspnea and increased respiratory infections. On auscultation, a "single S2 sound" can be heard, along with systolic ejection murmur and bounding peripheral pulses.

Diagnosis:

- Chest radiography shows cardiomegaly with increased pulmonary markings.
- Echocardiogram is the *gold standard*.
- Cardiac catheterization is rarely needed.

Treatment:

- Surgery repair is needed to avoid pulmonary hypertension and CHF.
- VSD and ASD are helpful and need to be kept open.

Tricuspid atresia

No tricuspid valve formation and no atrioventricular connection. Must have a persistent *foramen ovale* or ASD opening, for blood to transfer to the left heart.

Hx/PE: Babies are cyanotic soon after birth and on cardiac auscultation; a "single S1 sound" can be heard.

Diagnosis:

- EKG: left axis deviation.
- Chest radiography: reduced pulmonary markings.
- Echocardiogram (*diagnostic*): open foramen ovale open or ASD.

Treatment: PGE1 and surgery.

Third heart sounds

Third heart sounds are very common in children and some do not require further work-up.

Heart sounds/conditions that can be normal in neonates:

➤ Systolic murmurs.

➤ PDA can be normal, if do not last longer than 24 hours.

Note: Normal third heart sounds do not mean they do not need to be monitored.

Children with systolic murmurs

➤ Can happen in about 90% of all neonates and no further work-up is needed. They do need to be monitored.

➤ However, if diastolic murmur present then patient will need referral to a cardiologist and echocardiogram given for further evaluation.

Renovascular disease

The most frequent cause of secondary hypertension in young children.

Genetic defects

Down syndrome

Down syndrome is the *most common* trisomy syndrome (chromosome 21). Offer genetic screening to high-risk patients, history of previous Down syndrome births, or women aged >35 years.

Types:

➤ Meiotic non-disjunction: accounts for about 95% of all cases.

➤ **Robertsonian translocation**: accounts for about 5% of all cases.

➤ **Mosaic**: accounts for about 1%.

Note: Parents who have one child with Down syndrome have a 1% chance of having a second child with Down syndrome even if the mother is aged below 35 years.

Hx/PE: Speckling of iris, epicanthal folds, mental retardation, and small stature.

Diagnosis:

- Quadruple screening:
    - Increased hCG and inhibin A levels.
    - Decreased AFP and estradiol levels.
- Genetic screening for high risk patients, which needs to be consented.
    - If between 10 and 13 weeks of pregnancy, conduct chorionic villus sampling.
    - If between 15 and 20 weeks of pregnancy, then conduct amniocentesis.
- Echocardiogram: most common cardiac abnormality in Down syndrome is endocardial cushion defect.
- Hypothyroidism screening: can sample from heel pad but needs to be confirmed with blood draw.
- Rule out gastric pathology (TE and duodenal atresia).
- Rule out acute leukemia's later in life.
- Rule out diabetes.

Treatment: Treat underlying abnormalities and special needs.

Edwards syndrome

More commonly caused by nondisjunction, which causes a chromosomal abnormality characterized by the presence of extra genetic material on chromosome 18. Most die within the first few days-weeks of birth and only about 1% will live to 10 years of age (mainly mosaic [less severe]).

Hx/PE: Micrognathia, microcephaly, clenched first, rocker bottom feet, horseshoe kidney, and a median life span of 5-10 days.

Diagnosis:

- First quadruple screening: hCG, inhibin A, AFP, and estradiol levels are all decreased.
- Genetic testing (abnormal chromosome 18).
- If abnormal serum markers between 18 and 20 weeks, next step would be to perform an amniocentesis for confirmation.
- Screen with echocardiogram (e.g., VSD and ASD) and renal ultrasonography (horseshoe kidney).

Note:

- ✓Amniocentesis will need informed consent; order PTT, PT/INR, bleeding time, platelets, and cross-matching.
- ✓All invasive procedures need informed consent, exceptions are emergency situations.

Treatment: Treat underlying abnormalities.

Patau syndrome

A trisomy chromosomal abnormality with extra genetic material on chromosome 13. Risk of syndrome increases with maternal age and can be caused by nondisjunction, mosaic (better prognosis), and robertsonian. Death by 1 year of age in about 80%.

Hx/PE: Polydactyly, microcephaly, microphthalmia, cleft lip, and cleft palate.

Diagnosis:

- Quadruple screening: hCG, inhibin A, AFP, and estradiol levels; are not always useful in diagnosis since variable results.
- Genetic testing (abnormal chromosome 13).
- Screen with echocardiogram and renal ultrasonography.

Treatment: Varies from case to case. Cardiac surgery. Cleft lip surgery is usually performed at the age of 3 months.

Klinefelter syndrome

A genetic disorder resulting in two or more X chromosomes in males.

Risks: Infertility, undescended testicles, breast cancer (largest risk factor in males), and testicular cancer (germ cell).

Hx/PE: Tall, small testicles, non-tender gynecomastia, long extremities, and decreased IQ.

Diagnosis:

- LH (elevated), FSH (elevated), testosterone (low), and estrogen (elevated).
- **Karyotype** (XXY), with one Barr body (buccal smear).
  - The higher number of X chromosomes is associated with increased syndrome severity.

Treatment:

- May require special education.
- Testosterone replacement starting at age 11–12 years and surgery of undescended testicles may be required.

Turner syndrome

A genetic disorder where females are missing an X chromosome. Karyotype (XO).

Hx/PE: Gonadal dysgenesis, webbed neck, shield-like chest, widely spaced nipples, short stature, normal/low intelligence, no secondary sexual characteristics, and horseshoe kidney.

Diagnosis:

- Elevated FSH and LH levels, and low estradiol levels.
- Karyotype (XO). Buccal smear (no Barr bodies).
- Echocardiogram: rule out coarctation of the aorta.
- Negative progesterone challenge test because of lack of estrogen. However, in a progesterone and estrogen challenge test, the patient should bleed.

Treatment: Estrogen <u>plus</u> progesterone therapy (combination), growth hormone therapy, and anabolic steroids.

Note:

- ✓ Mother does <u>not</u> have an increased risk of having a second child with Turner syndrome.
- ✓ Patients with Turner syndrome have a low probability to become pregnant without assistance.
- ✓ Protect uterus with progesterone.

Phenylketonuria (PKU)

An autosomal recessive inborn error of metabolism of phenylalanine. A disorder, which involves *phenylalanine hydroxylase deficiency*.

<u>Risks</u> of developing **Tetralogy of Fallot.**

Hx/PE: Caucasian, shorter height than normal, low IQ, seizures, and "**musky odor**."

Diagnosis:

- Genetic screening (after feeding).
- Increased phenylalanine and decreased tyrosine levels.
- Commonly included in the newborn screening during the first week after birth.

Treatment:

- Increase tyrosine intake and reduce phenylalanine in the diet.
- Decrease intake of aspartame, egg whites, shrimp, elk meat, and soybean.

McCune-Albright syndrome

A genetic disorder of the skin, bones, and hormones. "**3Ps**" Peutz-Jegher syndrome, precocious puberty, pigmentation, and polyostotic fibrous dysplasia.

Fragile X syndrome

Genetic, X-linked, CGG triple repeat, anticipation, which is more common in males. Can present with ADHD, borderline, and mild/moderate mental retardation.

Hx/PE: Large ears, jaws, hands, and autism.

Diagnosis: Genetic testing (PCR): CGG triple repeat and methylation of FMR-1 gene.

Treatment: Special education, speech therapy, occupational therapy, and family counseling.

Cystic fibrosis (CF)

Autosomal recessive, chromosome 7, CFTR gene mutation, and CF508.

Risks: Associated with bronchiectasis, pneumonia, malabsorption, infertility, and meconium ileus (found in about 5-10% of patients).

Hx/PE: FTT, flatulence, increased respiratory infection, and malnutrition. Most common pathological factor in children for respiratory infections is actually *S. pneumonia* and not pseudomonas (gram-negative rod). Pseudomonas becomes more prevalent during teenage years. "Meconium ileus" is usually the earliest manifestation of CF (causes distal intestinal obstruction).

Diagnosis:

- Genetic testing and **sweat chloride test** (*best initial test* and *gold standard*) increased chloride.
- Electrolytes: decreased (NaCl) loss of sodium (hyponatremia) during sweat loss.
- Chest radiography: pneumonia secondary to *pseudomonas* and *S. pneumoniae.*
- Abdominal radiography: **meconium ileus** (bowel obstruction "ground glass").
- Gastrography enema.

Treatment:

- **Ivacaftor**: Helps restore the function of a mutated CF protein.

- Chest physical therapy (loosen impacted secretions), antibiotics, steroids, pancreatic enzymes, vitamin D, E, A, and K replacement, increase protein intake, medium-chained fatty acids, increase calorie intake, and vaccinations.
- Pulmonary pneumonia with IV tobramycin and ceftazidime <u>or</u> cefepime and amikacin.
- Meconium ileus: IV access, NPO, NG-tube, and possible surgery (bowel resection).
- Usually placed on life-long prophylactic antibiotics.

Pediatric gastroenterology

Choanal atresia

Obliteration or blockage of posterior nasal aperture/passage.

<u>Associated</u> with "CHARGE syndrome" <u>c</u>oloboma of the eye, <u>h</u>eart defects, <u>a</u>tresia of the choanae, <u>r</u>etardation of growth and development, <u>g</u>enital and urinary defects, and <u>e</u>ar anomalies and deafness.

Hx/PE: Symptoms can include cyanosis that worsens during breastfeeding and improves when infant cries. Atresia can be unilateral or bilateral.

Diagnosis:
- *Best initial test* is insertion of nose catheter.
- *Confirm* with head CT scan with contrast (which shows narrowing).

Treatment: Surgical intervention to perforate the membrane and reconnect the nostrils to the pharynx.

Tracheal esophageal fistula

Complications: "VACTERL": <u>v</u>ertebral abnormalities, <u>a</u>nal atresia, <u>c</u>ardiac defects, <u>t</u>racheal <u>e</u>sophagus, <u>r</u>enal abnormalities, and <u>l</u>imb abnormalities.

<u>Risks</u>: aspiration pneumonia, dehydration, malnutrition, and polyhydramnios.

Hx/PE: Drooling and choking on the first feed is a classic symptom of esophageal atresia. Esophageal atresia (most common abnormality).

Diagnosis:

- Chest radiography with NG-tube and bronchoscopy (*gold standard*).
- Echocardiogram to determine cardiac abnormalities.
- Baby gram to determine vertebral anomalies.

Treatment:

- *First step* is to place patient NPO and fluid hydration before surgery, since patient will become dehydrated.
- Surgical repair in two-step correction.
- Antibiotic coverage for aspiration pneumonia.
- Correct surgically other anomalies such as imperforated anus (**diverting colostomy**).

Congenital diaphragmatic hernia

A congenital malformation of the diaphragm. More common on the left side with decreased air entry on the left side. Usually full-term with pulmonary hypoplasia, pulmonary hypertension, and respiratory distress. High mortality rate with pulmonary hypertension and pulmonary hypoplasia.

Hx/PE: Bowel sounds are heard in the chest wall on physical exam and presents with respiratory distress.

Diagnosis:

- Ultrasonography can be diagnostic in utero.
- Chest radiography (postnatal) with presents of bowel in the hemithorax.

Treatment:

- *First step* is bowel rest (NPO), IV fluids, and NG-tube.
- Immediate intubation (low-pressure ventilation).
  - Do <u>not</u> bag mask the patient, as this can cause lung and stomach damage.
- Surgery (abdominal approach) required 2–4 days after birth to allow the lungs to reach maturity.

Gastroschisis

More common in premature infants. Caused secondary to the *neural crest* failure to migrate.

Complications: GI stenosis, intestinal atresia, and polyhydramnios.

Hx/PE: Occurs to the right of the umbilicus and has <u>no</u> peritoneal sac.

Diagnosis:

- Clinical diagnosis with physical examination (no peritoneal sac).
- Can suspect in utero if elevated MS-AFP levels and polyhydramnios.
- Need to rule out other GI problems.

Treatment:

- *First step* is delivery by C-section (as vaginal delivery has increased pressure).
- Keep infant on NG-tube, NPO, IV fluids, prophylactic antibiotics, and single-stage closer (only effective in 10%).
- **Emergency surgery** with **silo formation** (gradual).

Omphalocele

A type of abdominal wall defect where the bowels remain outside of the abdomen.

Complications: GI stenosis, intestinal atresia, polyhydramnios, and strongly associated with Edwards syndrome.

Hx/PE: The bowels are covered by the peritoneal sac.

Diagnosis:

- Clinical diagnosis.
- Can suspect in utero with elevated MS-AFP levels and polyhydramnios.
- Need to rule out other GI problems.

Treatment: Deliver by C-section. NPO, NG-tube, IV fluids, petroleum/gauze, and surgical closer.

Note: With omphalocele need to screen for trisomy 13, 18, and 21.

Pyloric stenosis

More common in first-born males that present with hypertrophy of the pyloric sphincter within 3-6 weeks of life. Can be associated to erythromycin use.

Hx/PE: "Projectile non-bilious vomitus."

Diagnosis:

- *Best initial test*: abdominal ultrasonography (*gold standard*); "olive shaped" mass.
- Electrolytes: hypochloremic, hypokalemic, and metabolic alkalosis (elevated bicarbonate levels).
- Barium study (pyloric beak).

Treatment:

- *First step*: NPO, NG-tube, and IV fluids.
- *Second step*: correct the electrolyte imbalance and metabolic alkalosis.
- *Third step*: **pyloromyotomy** (myotomy).

Note: In the case of a vomiting patient, consider aspiration pneumonia, metabolic alkalosis, dehydration, and electrolyte imbalance.

Duodenal atresia

Complete vs. partial obstruction. Associated with Down syndrome (highly) and annular pancreas.

Risks: GI and cardiac abnormalities, aspiration pneumonia, annular pancreas, malrotation, and imperforated anus.

Hx/PE: "Bilious vomiting" within 12 hours of birth.

Diagnosis:

- Abdominal radiography ("double bubble"), barium swallow, and upper endoscopy.
- Order: electrolytes, ABG, and chest x-ray (if suspicion aspiration pneumonia).

Note: "Double bubble" also found in annular pancreases and malrotation.

Treatment:

- Correct electrolytes, NG-tube (to decompress), NPO, and IV fluids.
- If aspiration pneumonia, treat with antibiotics.
- **Duodenostomy** (*definitive treatment*).

Volvulus

Medical emergency

Twisting of colon causing acute bowel obstruction and ischemia. Patient may present with history of bowel surgery. Highly associated with adhesions.

Hx/PE: Sudden colicky abdominal pain, bloody stool, bilious emesis, and abdominal distention.

Diagnosis:

- Gastrografin or abdominal radiography: "bird beak" appearance, no gas (distal), or normal appearance.
- Ultrasonography (sensitive) is determined by the skill of the ultrasonographer.
- *Study of choice*: upper endoscopy or colonoscopy.

Treatment:

- *Best initial therapy* is **emergency** endoscopic decompression, NPO, NG-tube, IV fluids, and antibiotic if suspicion of perforation or sepsis.
- May need surgical decompression and bowel removal, if necrotic.

Intussusception

Most common bowel obstruction in the first 2 years of life. Common at the ileocecal valve. Possible ischemia and commonly described as "sausage shape" or "target sign" on radiological findings.

Risks: adhesions, tumors, Meckel's, and abdominal surgery.

Hx/PE: Triad: abrupt colicky abdominal pain, vomiting, and blood per rectum; "black current-jelly like stool."

Diagnosis:

- *First step* is to stabilize patient.
- *Best initial test* is plain film or abdominal ultrasonography (target sign).
- **Air contrast enema** (*gold standard*) or bariun enema (rarely used).

Note: Barium enema is contraindicated in cases of perforation.

Treatment:

- Order: electrolytes (correct first), CBC (to rule out anemia), place on NG-tube (decompression), NPO, IV access, and IV fluids.
- Air contrast barium enema (often curative).
- Surgical resection (when air contrast or barium enema is not successful).
- Remove necrotic bowel (if needed).

Note:

✓ Most common complication of air contrast is bowel perforation.

✓ Air enema is both diagnostic and curative.

Malrotation

Most common is mid-gut malrotation. This can cause obstruction and ischemia owing to decrease blood supply to intestines.

Hx/PE: Patient can present with bilious vomitus.

Diagnosis: Barium enema (cecum on the left side of the abdomen) and abdominal radiography (no mass on the right side). If unstable, go straight to surgery.

Treatment: Laparotomy (**Ladd's procedure**).

Meckel's diverticulum

The <u>only</u> true congenital diverticulum; remnant of the omphalomesenteric (also called the **vitelline duct**).

Hx/PE: Commonly found in about 2% of the population, <2 years of age, 2 inches in length, 2 feet from the ileocecal valve, 2 types of tissue (pancreatic and gastric), and more common in males. "Painless bright red blood per rectum". Common complication is intussusception.

Diagnosis:

- Obtain CBC, electrolytes, ABG (if vomiting), and guaiac test.
- Use abdominal radiography to rule out perforation, followed by **Meckel's scintigraphy** (technetium 99c).

Treatment:

- *First steps*: NPO, NG-tube, IV fluids, and correct CBC (anemia).
- Surgical excision of diverticulum (**diverticulectomy**).

Hirschsprung's disease

A disorder characterized by absence of *ganglia* in the distal colon that results in intestinal obstruction.

Hx/PE: Constipation in neonates and no meconium passage within 24-48 hours is considered as Hirschsprung's until proven otherwise.

Diagnosis:
- *First step*, conduct physical examination (digital rectal examination) – tight sphincter and explosive stool.
- *Second step*, conduct anorectal manometry (*initial test*) and increase pressure during relaxation.
- *Third step*, conduct barium enema (proximal dilation) to support diagnosis.
- *Fourth step*, conduct full-thickness biopsy (no ganglion cells) of the rectal mucosa to confirm.

Treatment: Surgery and daily enemas while waiting for surgery can be used for daily cleaning.

Necrotizing enterocolitis (NEC)

NEC is the most common neonatal **GI emergency**. Premature infants (*greatest risk factor*).

Hx/PE: Feeding intolerance, metabolic acidosis, shock, peritonitis, bloody stools, local ischemia, abdominal distension, and infarction of the loops of the bowel. DIC risk.

Diagnosis:
- *Best initial test*: abdominal radiography (q6-hours) "**pneumatosis intestinalis**."
- CBC (low platelets and leukocytosis left shift), electrolytes, ABG, and blood culture.

Note: Low platelets in babies can represent sepsis.

Treatment:
- Correct CBC and electrolytes.
- Place: NPO, NG-tube, IV antibiotics (ampicillin, gentamycin, and metronidazole), IV fluids, and possible TPN.
- Surgery in cases of worsening abdominal radiography findings, necrosis, or perforation (reanastomosis).

Congenital umbilical hernias

Congenital weakness of the *umbilicus*. Highly associated with congenital hypothyroidism and 90% will close by the age of 3 years.

Diagnosis:
- Physical examination or abdominal ultrasonography.
- Rule out thyroid pathology (TSH/T4).

Treatment:
- If ≤1-2 cm, asymptomatic, and reducible can monitor till the age of 2–3 years.
- If persists after 4 years of age, surgical intervention is indicated.

Gastroesophageal reflux in child

Hx/PE: Infant or child spitting up formula or food after ingestion, chronic wheezing, and risk of aspiration pneumonia.

Diagnosis:
- Clinical diagnosis.
- *Optimal initial test* is esophageal pH monitoring, if need to confirm.
- If aspiration is suspected, perform chest radiography.

Treatment:
- Reassurance and formula thickening with rice cereal should be initiated.
- H_2-receptor blockers are *first-line drugs* in children because of safety.
- Surgery in severe cases of gastroesophageal reflux.

Note: PPIs is a more effective medication but first-line treatment in children are H_2 blockers.

Constipation in children

Can experience urinary retention, as colon impaction can exert pressure on the bladder.

Hx/PE: On physical examination: decreased bowel sounds, abdominal hard on palpation, and distended abdomen.

Diagnosis: Clinical diagnosis or abdominal radiography can be helpful. Rule out hypothyroidism.

Treatment:
- <u>Mild</u> constipation: dietary changes and magnesium hydroxide.
- <u>Severe</u> constipation (fecal impaction): enemas and suppositories.

Acute diarrhea in children

If no signs of dehydration, give normal age diet with <u>complex</u> carbohydrates, and diet low in sugar and fats (fats and sugar can exacerbate diarrhea).

<u>Normal considerations</u>:

- Infants (1-4 weeks) can stool 6 to 8 times a day (about one stool for each feeding).
- After 4 weeks of age, stools can decrease to 1-2 stools per day.

Obesity in children

More likely to be caused by overeating and less likely to be an underlying pathology.

Pediatric immunological disorders

Bruton's agammaglobulinemia

X-linked recessive more common in males, infections usually start after the age of 6 months (after there is decrease of the passive immunity from the mother). Presents with increased respiratory infections.

Hx/PE: Increased bacterial infections (encapsulated organisms).

Diagnosis: **Quantitative immunoglobulin levels** (measures immunoglobulin levels).

Treatment:

- Life-long immunoglobulins (usually monthly) and aggressive antibiotic management.
- No live vaccination because of immunosuppressed status, including MMR, influenza (nasal), and oral polio (sabin).

Common variable immunodeficiency

Characterized by low antibody levels and recurrent bacterial infections. Low levels of IgG (mainly), IgM (often), and IgA (often). Risk of developing lymphoma and autoimmune diseases.

Hx/PE: Signs and symptoms anytime between childhood and adulthood.

Diagnosis: Abnormal quantitative immunoglobulin levels.

Treatment: IVIGs (monthly) and antibiotics when needed.

IgA deficiency

Most common immunodeficiency with increased frequency of respiratory and GI tract infections.

Diagnosis: Quantitative immunoglobulin levels (low IgA levels).

Treatment: Antibiotics for infections.

Note: No IVIG treatment for IgA deficiency (controversial) because it can produce anti-IgA antibodies.

Wiskott-Aldrich syndrome

X-linked recessive, decreased IgM, and increased IgA. Has a 10% incidence of cancer particularly lymphoma and ALL. "WIPE": Wiskott, infection, platelets (low), and eczema.

Diagnosis: Physical examination (eczema), genetic testing, low IgM and elevated IgA, and CBC (low platelets).

Treatment:

- Supportive treatment (patients rarely live to adulthood).
- IVIGs and antibiotics.
- Severe cases: bone marrow transplant.

Chronic granulomatous disease (CGD)

X-linked or AR, deficiency in NADPH oxidase, no superoxide production, and increased catalase-producing organisms.

Diagnosis:

- **Nitroblue tetrazolium test**: checks for the presence of functional catalase.
- Absolute neutrophil count.
- Genetic testing.

Treatment:

- INF-gamma (decreases incidence).
- TMP-SMX (prophylaxis), bone marrow transplant, and/or gene therapy.

DiGeorge syndrome

Associated with tetany (decreased calcium levels), decreased T-cell count, CATCH-22, defective thymus and parathyroid gland. Increased viral, atypical bacteria, and fungal infections (especially *Pneumocystis jiroveci* and *P. carinis*).

Hx/PE: "CATCH": cardiac abnormalities, abnormal facies, thymic dysfunction, calcium abnormalities, and hypoparathyroidism.

Diagnosis:
- Electrolytes: most importantly ionized calcium (hypocalcemia).
- **Absolute lymphocyte count**.
- Echocardiogram: heart defects.
- Chest radiography: no hypoplastic thymic shadow.
- PCR genotyping: *most specific diagnosis*.

Treatment: Correct low calcium (life-long calcium and vitamin D), infections (antibiotics), heart defects (surgery), PCP prophylaxis (SMP-TMX), bone marrow transplant, and thymus transplant (severe cases).

Ataxia-telangiectasia

Autosomal recessive, cerebellar ataxia (poor coordination), oculocutaneous telangiectasia (dilated blood vessels), and decreased IgA and IgE levels. Absent or mutation of **ATM protein**.

Risk of non-Hodgkin's lymphoma, leukemia, and GI tract cancer.

Diagnosis: Genetic testing and quantitative immunoglobulin levels (low IgA).

Treatment: Possible IVIGs and for the ataxia requires physical and occupational therapy.

Severe combined immunodeficiency (SCID)

Also known as bubble baby disease. Decreased B-cells and T-cells, which can lead to increase risk of all the subtypes of infections including fungal, viral, atypical, and typical bacterial infections. Not diagnosed until about 6 months of age when passive immunity fades.

Diagnosis: Quantitative immunoglobulin levels and absolute lymphocyte count.

Treatment:
- PCP prophylaxis (SMP-TMX plus folic acid).
- IVIGs, bone marrow transplant, and stem cell transplant.
- Research is focusing on genetically altering the genetic sequence.

Note: Stem cell transplant treatment can lead to a high incidence of leukemia in the SCID population.

Leukocyte adhesion deficiency (LAD)

Autosomal recessive, which causes recurrent infection secondary to decreased chemotaxis of leukocytes (*adhesion defect*), decreased pus formation, and decreased inflammation.

Hx/PE: Delayed separation of the umbilical cord and omphalitis.

Diagnosis: WBC with differentials: <u>High</u> WBC count but not effective (no pus formation and minimal inflammation).

Treatment: Bone marrow transplant is *curative*. Advancements in gene therapy are positive.

Chediak–Higashi syndrome

Autosomal recessive, with a defect in the **lysosomal trafficking regulator protein**, which causes a decrease in phagocytosis.

Hx/PE: <u>Triad</u>: ocular albinism, neuropathy, and neutropenia.

Diagnosis: WBC with differentials: neutropenia. Bone marrow smear: "**giant inclusion bodies**."

Treatment: Bone marrow transplant and antibiotics.

C1 esterase deficiency

An autosomal dominate disorder where the system is <u>not</u> able to suppress the complement system. This disrupts the flow of fluids because of the exacerbated inflammation.

Hx/PE: Can be mistaken for an anaphylaxis reaction. Presents with angioedema (lasts 24–74 hours), splenic dysfunction, and life-threatening pulmonary edema.

Diagnosis: **Total complement activity** (CH50) and **purified C1 esterase**.

Treatment: **C1 inhibitor concentrate** or FFP ([alternative] contains C1 inhibitor).

Terminal complement deficiency

Affects the complement membrane attack complex with deficiency of C5-C9. Decreased membrane attack complex (MAC), can increase the risk of meningococcal and gonococcal infections.

Hx/PE: In case of <u>disseminated</u> gonorrhea infection, rule out this deficiency.

Diagnosis: Total complement activity (CH50).

Treatment:

- In cases of gonococcal infections, it is difficult to obtain a culture; so culture from multiple locations (mouth, urethral, anus, and cervix).
- Meningococcal vaccination and antibiotic treatment, as needed for infections.

Note: There is no vaccination for gonorrhea.

Pediatric infectious diseases

Bronchiolitis

Inflammation of the bronchioles. Most commonly caused by RSV (about 70% of cases) and parainfluenza virus. More common during fall and winter. Causes air trapping and over inflation.

Risk factors include contact with sick individuals and second-hand smoke.

Hx/PE: Mild fever, rhinorrhea, cough, expiratory wheezing, and hyperresonance.

Diagnosis:

- Clinical diagnosis (no further examinations needed usually).
- *Optimal initial test*: chest radiography (hyperinflated, flattened diaphragm, atelectasis, and interstitial infiltrates).
  - Chest x-ray: can lead to over diagnosis of pneumonia and antibiotic use.
  - Chest x-ray will be needed if condition does not resolve or symptoms last >10 days (to rule out pneumonia).

Types of testing:
  - **NP-swab culture** (used to rule out, viral, fungal, and bacteria involvement): works by introducing a sterile cotton swab through the nostril.
  - **Rapid strep test** (used to rule out bacterial infection): the

advantage is that results are obtained within minutes but is not as specific as throat culture.

- **Throat culture**: more *specific* than Rapid strep test but can take a few days to get the results.

Treatment:

- In cases of mild disease: only supportive treatment.
- In cases of moderate or severe disease: give fluids, oxygen, and hospitalize.
- **Ribavirin**: consider in high-risk children (heart or lung disease).

Note: Also hospitalize if <3 months of age, born premature (<34 weeks), PaO_2 <95%, toxic appearing, or dehydrated.

Croup (laryngotracheobronchitis)

Croup is an acute viral upper respiratory infection caused mainly by parainfluenza, RSV, or influenza.

Hx/PE: Upper respiratory symptoms, inspiratory stridor, and "barking cough."

Diagnosis: Clinical diagnosis or if needed; order pulse oximetry, NP-swab culture, and AP neck radiography ("steeple sign") with subglottic narrowing.

Treatment:

- *Mild*: (self-limiting) if oxygen levels less than 92% give humidified oxygen, cold mist, and fluids.
- *Moderate*: oxygen, fluids, nebs, steroids, and racemic epinephrine.
- *Severe*: hospitalize, steroids, and give **racemic epinephrine** via a nebulizer.

Prevention: Yearly influenza vaccine (more commonly given during fall).

- Do not give IM influenza vaccination, if child is aged below 6 months.
- If using nasal influenza spray (live vaccination), do not administer to children aged below 2 years.

Epiglottitis
Medical emergency

Epiglottitis is an inflammation of the epiglottis most commonly caused by *Haemophilus influenzae* type B.

Hx/PE: High fever, difficulty breathing, swallowing, "drooling," difficulty speaking, stridor, nasal flaring, and retractions. Patient may find relief in "sniffing dog position" (neck hyperextended).

Diagnosis: *First step*: transfer to ICU and perform endotracheal intubation, and then obtain <u>lateral</u> neck radiography "thumb print." Fiberoptic bronchoscopy (*gold standard*).

Treatment: STAT intubation (by ENT doctor or anesthesiologist) and IV ceftriaxone.

Prevention: *H. influenzae* type b vaccination (Hib) can be given at the age of 2, 4, 6, and 12 months.

Retropharyngeal abscess

More common in infants and young children and usually involves deeper tissues.

Hx/PE: Neck stiffness, dysphagia, drooling, and cervical lymphadenopathy (unilateral). Hard to diagnose with physical examination.

Diagnosis: Lateral radiography and contrast neck CT scan (*most specific test*).

Treatment:

- Incision and drainage (often involving tonsillectomy) and high-dose antibiotics.
- Intubation, if obstruction.

Pertussis (whooping cough)

A respiratory infection caused by *Bordetella pertussis* that is <u>highly</u> infectious and can be life threatening. Harsh coughing can cause subconjunctival hemorrhages.

Stages:

> 1st: catarrhal.

> 2nd: paroxysmal.

> 3rd: convalescent.

Diagnosis: Diagnosis is mainly clinical but can order: CBC (high WBC), pulse oximetry, ABG, NP swab culture, throat culture, and chest radiography.

Treatment:

- Use erythromycin (10-14 days) or azithromycin (3-5 days).
- Treat individuals with close contact with same regiment.
- No school until 5 days after starting antibiotics.

Prevention: DTaP ×5 (2 months, 4 months, 6 months, 1 years, and 4 years).

Meningitis in children

Bacterial meningitis is a **medical emergency**.

Common agents: GBS, *listeria*, *E. coli*, *S. pneumonia*, and *N. meningitis*.

Hx/PE: Headache, fever, FTT, positive Kerning and Brudzinski's sign, petechial rash, photophobia, and papillary edema.

Bacterial tetrad: Fever, nuchal rigidity, photophobia, and headache.

Diagnosis:

- If clear diagnosis and signs of ICP then administer IV antibiotics.
- Head CT scan w/o contrast should be done before lumbar puncture, if the patient presents with focal neurologic findings, papillary edema, new seizure, or AMS.
  - Next step after head CT scan, if no contraindications, is lumbar puncture (*most specific test*).
- Blood culture should be done before antibiotics, if stable.
- Lumbar puncture should also technically be performed before administering IV antibiotics, but antibiotics may be administered first in cases where the patient is unstable or if

a lumbar puncture is scheduled within 2 hours of antibiotic administration.

Note: Time is important for meningitis and STAT orders are required.

Treatment:

- Neonates (<1 month): amoxicillin plus cefotaxime or gentamicin.
- Children (>1 month): ceftriaxone and vancomycin.
- Adolescents and teens: ceftriaxone and vancomycin.

Chemoprophylaxis: **rifampin** (for *N. meningitis* and HiB).

Urinary tract infection in children

Common in males below 1 year of age and females during toilet training (wiping from back to front). More common in women than males because of shorter urethra. Most common cause of UTI is *E. coli* (gram-negative rod). A major risk factor in children is **vesicoureteral reflux** (abnormal urinary backflow from the bladder).

Hx/PE: Fever, dysuria, polyuria, and nocturia.

Diagnosis:

- *Initial test* (urinalysis) and *most accurate test* (urine culture).
- In patients aged <u>below</u> 2 years of age, >2 UTIs, family history, male, or causative organism is other than *E. coli*, patient will need renal/bladder ultrasonography.
  - If abnormal ultrasonography then a **voiding cystourethrogram** (VCUG) is indicated.
- Follow-up urinalysis 1 month after treatment and regular assessments for the next 2 years.

Treatment:

- If child is ≤24 months and first UTI, should treat for ≥7 days.
- In cases of <u>non-toxic</u> appearance (**cystitis**), increase oral hydration and oral antibiotics (amoxicillin or SMX-TMP).
  - Do not give SMX-TMP or nitrofurantoin, if aged below 1 month.
- In case of <u>toxic</u> appearance or suspicion of <u>pyelonephritis</u>:

hospitalization and IV antibiotics (ceftriaxone or ampicillin plus gentamicin).

- <u>Vesicoureteral reflux</u>: use prophylaxis nitrofurantoin or SMP-TMX for the first year after diagnosis.

- Antibiotic rules for children:

  - Aged below 1 month, do not give TMP-SMX or nitrofurantoin.

  - Aged below 8 years, do not give tetracycline's (doxycycline).

  - Aged below 16 years, do not give quinolones.

Note:

✓ Remember, if the <u>mother</u> has pyelonephritis during pregnancy, give IV amoxicillin and gentamycin.

✓ Toxic appearance or pyelonephritis requires IV antibiotics.

✓ Non-toxic cystitis can be treated with oral antibiotics.

Erythema infectiosum (parvovirus B19)

Also known as **fifth disease** or **slapped cheek**. Pregnant women should avoid contact with children with fifth disease in the first trimester (spontaneous miscarriage). Can lead to hemolytic anemia, hydrops fetalis, and aplastic crisis (sickle cell anemia and spherocytosis).

Hx/PE: Low-grade fever, cold-like symptoms, and <u>then</u> rash begins a few days after symptoms reside. Not contagious once rash begins.

Diagnosis: Clinical diagnosis or CBC should be performed to determine hematocrit levels.

Treatment:

- Usually self-limiting.

- Supportive treatment with antipyretics (acetaminophen <u>or</u> NSAIDs) and temperature monitoring.

- If **aplastic crisis** develops, patient may require transfusions.

Note: In erythema infectiosum once the rash appears, patients are non-infectious and can return to school or daycare.

Measles

Highly contagious viral infection caused by the measles virus (paramyxovirus family). Rare presentation: **subacute sclerosing panencephalitis.**

Hx/PE: <u>Tetrad</u>: "**4Cs**" conjunctivitis, cough, coryza (rhinitis), and **Koplik's spots** (whitish spots on the buccal mucosa, is *diagnostic*).

Diagnosis: Clinical diagnosis (fever with at least one clinical picture [conjunctivitis, cough, or coryza]) or blood culture (PCR).

Treatment: Supportive (self-limiting): acetaminophen (fever), fluids, and rest.

<u>Prevention</u>: MMR vaccination given at 1 and 4 years of age.

Mumps

Infection caused by the mumps virus (paramyxovirus family). Transmission is via airborne droplets, saliva, and direct contact.

Hx/PE: "**POM POMs**": <u>p</u>arotitis (mainly), <u>o</u>rchitis, and <u>m</u>eningoencephalomyelitis.

Diagnosis: Clinical diagnosis or blood testing (PCR).

Treatment:
- Supportive: acetaminophen, fluids, and rest.
- Can return to school or work one week after diagnosis.

<u>Prevention</u>: MMR vaccination between 1 and 4 years of age.

Rubella

Infection caused by the rubella virus (togavirus family). Can cause cataracts, glaucoma, deafness, encephalitis, decrease platelets, and PDA. Rubella is part of the "TORCH" screening.

Hx/PE: Usually rash starts in the face and spreads distally. Spares palms and soles.

Diagnosis: Clinical diagnosis. If mother is pregnant will need further work-up.

Treatment: Supportive: acetaminophen, fluids, and rest.

Prevention:

- MMR vaccination given at the age of 1 and 4 years.
- Not recommended to give to mother during pregnancy.

Roseola

Caused by (HHV-6 and 7). Increased risk of **febrile seizures** (no work-up needed for simple febrile seizures). Usually, children below 6 years of age experience febrile seizures.

Hx/PE: Rash followed by fever (>40°C).

Diagnosis: Clinical diagnosis (rash and fever never at the same time).

Treatment: Usually no treatment needed. Acetaminophen or NSAIDs can be helpful to decrease fever but no studies show they prevent febrile seizures.

Varicella

Caused by herpes virus and known as **chickenpox**, which is more common in children. Infants <10 months of age have a 25% mortality rate.

Risk of developing: meningoencephalitis.

Hx/PE: Patient presents with mild fever, painful lesions, and pruritus. Lesions appear as vesicular teardrop shaped lesions. There is epidermal pain before lesions become present and lesions can appear at different stages.

Stages:

- 1ˢᵗ: erythema.
- 2ⁿᵈ: papules.
- 3ʳᵈ: vesicular (contagious 24 hours before vesicle formation).

➤ 4th: crusting lesion (end of cycle and non-contagious).

Diagnosis:

- Clinical diagnosis or can be confirmed with Tzanck smear (multi-nucleated giant cells).
- *Most specific test* is HSV PCR.

Treatment:

- Supportive treatment and pain control.
- Congenital varicella (neonate): IV acyclovir and **VariZIG** (purified human immunoglobulin with anti-varicella antibodies).
- Maternal varicella: treated in the same way as congenital varicella.
- Toddlers: for patients aged <10 months, immunosuppressed patients, and severe or disseminated disease, acyclovir is recommended.
- Children: varicella is self-limiting. For patients aged >13 years, acyclovir is recommended.

Prevention: Varicella vaccination (live vaccine) given at the age of 1 and 4 years.

Zoster

Viral infection caused by the herpes virus and is also known as shingles. Not common in children and is a reactivation disease with dermal distribution that tends to affect the sensory nerves.

Risks: encephalitis, conjunctivitis, GBS, pneumonia, and TTP.

Hx/PE: Normally presents with malaise, fever, and a painful localized rash with blisters.

Diagnosis: Clinical diagnosis and if needed can confirm with Tzanck smear (multi-nucleated giant cells) or PCR.

Treatment:

- Oral or IV acyclovir in cases of immunosuppression. Topical acyclovir can help with pain in mild cases.
- Pain treatment options: Calamine, opioids, capsaicin, steroids, and gabapentin.

Hand-foot-mouth disease

Highly contagious disease most commonly caused by Coxsackie A virus. Risk of developing encephalitis.

Hx/PE: <u>Painful</u> oral ulcers and rashes on the hands and feet.

Diagnosis: Clinical diagnosis or throat culture.

Treatment: No cure, self-limiting but can give acetaminophen for fever and pain.

Kawasaki disease

An autoimmune disease mainly seen in children that causes acute vasculitis (inflammation of blood vessels) and is a leading cause of acquired heart disease in the United States.

Hx/PE: "CRASH and BURN": <u>c</u>onjunctivitis, <u>r</u>ash (hands and feet), coronary <u>a</u>neurysm, <u>s</u>trawberry tongue, and <u>h</u>eat with a body temperature of >40°C for 5 days.

Diagnosis:

- <u>Subacute phase</u>: ESR (high), CRP levels (high), CBC (thrombocytosis, starts 2 weeks after fever).
- <u>Chronic phase</u>: starts after all symptoms disappear and lasts until the ESR normalizes.
- If left untreated, there is a risk of coronary aneurysm or MI.

Treatment:

- *First*, give IVIG (prevents coronary artery aneurysm) and high-dose aspirin (decreases fever, pain, thrombosis, and inflammation).
  - After fever breaks follow with low dose aspirin for 6 weeks.
- Add warfarin, if there is high risk of thrombosis.
- Echocardiogram: long-term management by cardiologist.

Note:

✓ Steroid use for Kawasaki disease has <u>not</u> been shown to be affective and can lead to elevated risk of coronary artery aneurysm.

✓ Aspirin can be associated with **Reye's syndrome**.

Cerebral palsy

Cerebral palsy is a disorder of movement, muscle tone, and posture.

Types:

➤ Pyramidal (spastic).

➤ Extrapyramidal (dyskinetic).

Hx/PE: Mental retardation, visual impairment, hearing loss, skeletal malformation, communication disorder, seizures, poor growth, feeding problems, constipation, toe walking, "**scissor walking**", spasticity, and contractures.

Diagnosis: Clinical diagnosis.

- Infants: head ultrasonography and EEG.
- Children: head MRI and EEG.

Treatment: Physical therapy, occupational therapy, behavioral therapy, speech therapy, and special education. Contractures (surgical release). Spasticity (baclofen). Seizure (anti-seizure medications).

Pediatric fever

Febrile seizures

Commonly associated with roseola (HHV-6 and HHV-7). Diagnosis of exclusion caused by high fever, more commonly in children aged below 6 years. No risk or very low risk of developing epilepsy in cases of febrile seizures.

➤ **Simple seizures**: duration lasts <15 minutes and only one seizure within 24 hours (no work-up needed).

➤ **Complex seizures**: duration lasts >15 minutes or more than one seizure within 24 hours (always needs work-up).

Diagnosis:

- In most cases, no work-up is needed.

- Important to evaluate the source of the fever.

- <12 months of age, suspicion of meningitis, <u>or</u> complex seizure then order septic work-up:

  - Work-up may include head MRI, EEG, and lumbar puncture.

Treatment:

- Acetaminophen or NSAIDs (helps with fever but no studies show that they prevent future seizures).

- Diazepam or barbiturates are helpful for uncontrolled seizures.

- There is a 30% chance of developing a second febrile seizure but very low or no likelihood of developing epilepsy.

Pediatric cancers

Leukemia

*Full list of all leukemia types in the Hematology section of the *In Your Pocket* series.

A type of cancer that usually develops in the bone marrow resulting in the production of a high number of underdeveloped WBCs; known as, blasts or leukemia cells. There are many types of leukemia including ALL, AML, CLL, and CML.

Diagnosis: CBC with peripheral blood smear: WBC (high, normal, or low), H/H (low), and platelets (low). Specific markers will depend on suspicion. Bone marrow aspiration (*gold standard*) but rarely done.

Treatment: Chemotherapy is the *treatment of choice*. Consider radiation and bone marrow transplant.

Note: Chemotherapy can cause hyperuremia, which can be prevented with fluids, diuretics, allopurinol, and urine alkalization.

Neuroblastoma

Neuroblastoma is the third most common neoplasm in the pediatric population. A neuroendocrine tumor arising from a neural crest origin of the CNS. Usually involves the adrenal glands. Can develop in nerve tissues in the chest, neck, and abdomen. Associated with **N-myc**.

Hx/PE: If the tumor is located in the adrenal gland can manifest as a painless abdominal mass tumor that secretes norepinephrine. On rare occasion, might experience opsoclonus-myoclonus-ataxia ("dancing feet").

Diagnosis:

- CBC, electrolytes (usually normal), BUN/Cr ratio, urinalysis, homovanillic acid, vanillylmandelic acid, and 24-hour catecholamine levels.

- Abdominal ultrasonography, abdominal CT scan, mIBG scan, and FNA (blue tumor).

Note: Tumors in neuroblastoma <u>can</u> cross-midline unlike Wilms' tumor.

Treatment: Control blood pressure, tumor excision, radiation, and chemotherapy.

Wilms' tumor

Renal tumor with a possible mutation of the **WT1 gene** on chromosome 11 (other genes can be involved). Involvement of "WAGR": Wilms' tumor, aniridia, genitourinary abnormalities, and mental retardation. Might present with hypertension (more common in bilateral involvement). Hypertension in children needs investigation of Wilms' tumor and neuroblastoma.

Hx/PE: Abdominal pain, abdominal distension, weight loss, and hypertension.

Diagnosis:

- CBC, electrolytes, BUN/Cr ratio, and urinalysis (hematuria in about 20%).

- *Best initial test*: abdominal ultrasonography.

- Genetic testing and abdominal CT scan.
- Renal biopsy is not typically performed because of seeding risk.

Note: Wilms' tumor does <u>not</u> cross the midline.

Treatment: First control blood pressure and then perform resection or nephrectomy, followed by radiation and chemotherapy.

<u>Screening</u>: Children with minor trauma and microhematuria will need to be screened for congenital anomalies. Would also need to screen IQ testing and ophthalmic examination.

Ewing's sarcoma

Bone or soft tissue tumor (blue tumor) more common in males. Associated with chromosome translocation of 11:22 and primitive neuroectodermal. Commonly found in pelvis, humerus, or tibia.

Hx/PE: Bone pain (worse at night), fractures, swelling, and weight loss.

Diagnosis:

- WBC (elevated), alkaline phosphatase (elevated), and ESR (elevated).
- Bone radiography (lamellated or "onion-skin"), bone scan, and bone MRI.
- Genetic testing (*specific test*).

Treatment: Multi-drug chemotherapy and radiation (more useful for localized tumor). Excision usually done after a few trails of chemotherapy, which decreases tumor size.

Osteosarcoma

A type of bone tumor more common in children and usually located in the <u>distal</u> femur. Associated with Paget's disease and retinoblastoma.

Hx/PE: Bone pain (worse at night), fractures, swelling, and weight loss.

Diagnosis:

- WBC (elevated), ESR (elevated), and alkaline phosphatase (elevated).

- Radiography ("**sunburst**" appearance), bone scan, and bone MRI.
- *Specific testing*: genetic testing and bone biopsy.

Treatment: Chemotherapy and radiation. Excision usually done after chemotherapy, which decrease tumor size.

Von Hippel-Lindau syndrome (VHL)

Genetic disease caused by mutation of the Von Hippel-Lindau tumor suppressor gene on chromosome 3. Associated with pancreatic cysts, renal carcinomas, pheochromocytomas, and hemangioblastomas.

Diagnosis: Genetic testing (*most specific*), BUN/Cr ratio, urinalysis, urine culture, renal ultrasonography, head MRI, and 24-hour urine catecholamine testing.

Treatment: No cure for VHL. Treat underlying pathology.

Sarcoma botryoides

Rare vaginal malignancy in young girls.

Hx/PE: Most common clinical finding is vaginal bleeding.

Diagnosis: Physical examination: presents as bloody vaginal discharge, with "**grape-like**" masses protruding through the urethra or vagina.

Treatment: Multi-drug chemotherapy, radiation, and surgery.

Pediatric nutrition deficiency

Rickets

Caused by dietary deficiency in vitamin D (more commonly), calcium, or phosphorus. Which causes weakness of the bones and susceptibility to fractures. Ulnar/radial bowing and a "**waddling gait**" due to tibia/femoral bowing. Bowlegs are a characteristic sign.

Hx/PE: Tetany, bone tenderness, teeth abnormalities, and growth disturbance.

Diagnosis:

- CBC (possible anemia)and electrolytes: low ionized calcium and phosphate. Alkaline phosphatase can be elevated.

- Chest radiography: hypodensity of bones. "**Rachitic rosary-like**" appearance of the costochondral joints.

Treatment:

- Supplement with vitamin D, phosphate, calcium, and sunlight.

- Severe cases may require surgery for severely deformed bones.

Note: Vitamin D helps with calcium absorption.

Common vitamin deficiencies in children

➤ **Iron deficiency**: risk of deficiency during growing stages (2 years, 5 years, and 11 years), heavy menstruation in females during puberty, malnutrition, and heavy bleeding.

- Breast milk does <u>not</u> have enough iron after 6 months of life (can cause iron deficient anemia).

➤ **Calcium deficiency**: breastfeeding neonates need to receive vitamin D supplementation (human breast milk is insufficient), which helps absorb calcium. Can also occur during growth stages and secondary to malnutrition.

➤ **Folic acid deficiency**: malnutrition in growing children, low intake of vegetables, and certain medications.

➤ **B12 deficiency**: vegan mothers need supplementation during breastfeeding. Also can be caused by malnutrition, Crohn's disease, growing children, certain medications, and lack of animal products and proteins in diet.

Pediatric genetic disease

Vitamin D-dependent rickets (type I)

A genetic disorder causing weakening and softening of the bone tissue. Abnormal regulation of **1-α-hydroxylation enzyme** in the kidneys (normal or high 25(OH)D and low 1,25(OH)2D levels).

Diagnosis: Low phosphate, low calcium, and increased alkaline phosphate.

Treatment: Sunlight and diet rich in calcium and vitamin D.

Prader-Willi syndrome

Deletion of gene locus, chromosome 15q11-13. Paternally inherited.

Hx/PE: Hypotonia, obesity, mental retardation, behavioral issues, binge eating, short height, hypogonadism, and "almond-shaped eyes."

Diagnosis: Genetic testing (*mainstream testing*) deletion of 15q11q13.

Treatment: Special education, speech therapy, physical therapy, and growth hormone.

Friedreich's ataxia

Autosomal recessive disease, which causes damage to the nervous system. Associated with trinucleotide repeat (GAA), atrophy of the cervical spinal cord and cerebellum. Loss of vibratory and position sensation.

Hx/PE: Gait disturbance, visual impairment, loss of coordination, hearing impairment, and slurred speech. Does not cause cognitive dysfunction.

Diagnosis: Genetic testing (GAA triple repeats).

Treatment: Stem cell therapy (short lived), physical therapy, speech therapy, and occupational therapy.

Henoch-Schonlein purpura

A systemic vasculitis with IgA deposits on vessels, more common in males and is most common cause of non-thrombocytopenic purpura in children. Usually occurs a few weeks after a viral infection. Children might have thrombocytosis. Can present with acute renal failure.

Hx/PE: Fever, lower-extremity palpable purpura, edema, arthritis, and abdominal pain.

Diagnosis: CBC (can show elevated platelets), electrolytes, urinalysis (RBCs/proteins), BUN/Cr ratio (elevated), ESR (elevated), and skin biopsy (rarely done).

Treatment: Self-limiting and supportive treatment: NSAIDs (abdominal pain) and steroids (if given early in the course). Can consider heparin and warfarin.

Sudden infant death syndrome

Also known as crib death. Death is sudden and unexpected.

Risk factors: Low birth weight, teenage pregnancy, smoking habit in parents, sleeping position on the stomach or side, and genetics (more common in males).

Diagnosis: Diagnosis of exclusion and can support diagnosis if diffused intrathoracic petechiae are observed during autopsy. Always keep in mind child abuse.

Treatment: Baby should sleep on their back with no toys in the sleeping area (for first 2–4 months). Breastfeeding is preventive. Offer emotional support to family with counseling.

Pediatric ophthalmology

Amblyopia

A disorder of sight also known as lazy eye. This is caused by misalignment of the eye/s leading to suppression of images from the misaligned eye by the brain and increasing the risk of visual loss. Usually unilateral.

Strabismus

Also known as **cross eye**, and is the most common cause of amblyopia. Can be normal until 3 months of age (can outgrow strabismus).

Diagnosis: **Corneal light test** (asymmetrical) and Snellen chart.

Treatment:
- Corrective lens and occlusion of the dominant eye (normal eye).
- Surgery is the last resort.

Leukocoria

An abnormal white papillary reflex coming from the retina of the eye. Need to rule out retinoblastoma or congenital cataracts.

Diagnosis: **Red light reflex** (screening test needs to done before discharge) with an abnormal pupil that appears white.

Treatment: Treat underlying cause: infection, retinoblastoma, or cataracts, etc.

Retinoblastoma (RB)

A fast-growing cancer of the retina, associated with chromosome 13 (called RB1). This cancer needs to be treated as soon as possible, as it can cause blindness and even death.

Hx/PE: Red light reflex: an abnormal red light reflex (pupil appears white), is retinoblastoma until proven otherwise.

Diagnosis:
- Genetic testing: loss of function of tumor suppressor Rb gene on locus 13q chromosome.

- Will need full work-up with head CT scan and MRI.

Treatment: Needs immediate ophthalmologic examination with pupillary dilation under anesthesia to assess extent of disease progression.

Dacryostenosis

Stricture or narrowing of a *lacrimal duct*.

Hx/PE: Usually unilateral and painless with increased tears and mucus.

Diagnosis: History and physical examination (possible palpable mass).

Treatment:
- Nasolacrimal massage if <1 year.
- **Nasolacrimal duct probing** (dilating duct) if >1 year.

Note: Often resolves during the first year of life on its own.

Pediatric poisoning

Reye's syndrome

Secondary to aspirin intake in the pediatric population. Patients can present with **acute hepatic encephalopathy** with high ammonia levels. One of the rare approved uses of aspirin in the pediatric population is for Kawasaki disease (as the benefits outweigh the risks in this case).

Diagnosis: Blood glucose (may be low), BUN/Cr ratio (elevated) ammonium levels (high), AST (high), ALT (high), PT (high), PTT (high), platelets (low), amylase (high), lipase (high), and ABG (respiratory alkalosis at <u>early</u> stages and metabolic acidosis at <u>later</u> stages of aspirin toxicity).

Treatment: Stop aspirin, monitor respiration and breathing, monitor for seizures, and AMS.

Lead poisoning

Can cause <u>sideroblastic anemia</u>, decreased MCV (<80), increased iron levels, impaired intelligence, encephalopathy, gingival lines, seizures, and confusion. The greatest risk of development in children with lead poisoning is cognitive impairment.

Hx/PE: More commonly seen in children living in a house built in the 1950s (as lead was introduced in the paint products during this period). Patients present to hospital with altered mental status.

Diagnosis:
- Obtain blood lead levels:
  - If 10–14 µg/dL, retest in 3 months.
  - If 15–19 µg/dL, retest in 2 months.
  - If 20–44 µg/dL, retest in 1 week.
- MCV (<80), iron (high), and lead levels (high).
- Peripheral blood smear ("basophilic stippling").
- If levels are obtained by capillary test, confirm with <u>venous</u> blood draw.

Treatment: Treatment depends on the levels:
- <45 µg/dL: retesting depends on above levels.
- 45–69 µg/dL: inpatient EDTA <u>or</u> outpatient DMSA (succimer).
- >70 µg/dL: hospitalize; EDTA and BAL.

Pediatric congenital disorders

Thymic shadow

Can be found in children on radiography and is caused by a thymic shadow. Thymic shadow is known as the "sail sign" and is a normal finding on radiography until the age of 2 years. After this age, consider left lower lobe collapse.

Nasal polyps

Usually secondary to chronic inflammation/congestion and most commonly caused by allergic reactions.

Hx/PE: Nontender movable nodules, nasal wheezing, runny nose, and sneezing.

Diagnosis: Nasal endoscopy and biopsy (if cancer is suspected).

Treatment:
- Usually treated with nasal topical corticosteroid spray or nasal decongestants.
- Systemic steroids if unsuccessful, followed by surgical intervention (endoscopic surgery), if needed.

Thyroglossal duct cyst

Generally benign fibrous cyst that arises from the *primitive thyroglossal duct*. This cyst is found in the <u>midline</u> and is connected to the tongue.

Hx/PE: Can develop oral obstruction, dysphagia, and difficulty swallowing.

Diagnosis:
- TSH and FT4 levels (to rule out thyroid dysfunction).
- Neck radiography, neck ultrasound, thyroid scan, and FNA.

Treatment: Surgical removal when becomes problematic or cosmetic reasons.

Brachial cleft cyst

Remnant of embryonic development. Arises from the lateral part of the neck and caused by failure of obliteration of the <u>second</u> brachial cleft.

Hx/PE: A mass in front of the sternomastoid muscle that can be fluctuant. Usually asymptomatic.

Diagnosis:

- TSH and FT4 levels (to rule out thyroid dysfunction).
- Neck radiography, ultrasound, and MRI.

Treatment: Surgical excision if large (keep in mind the structures that can be problematic post-surgery).

Cystic hygroma

A benign abnormal formation of the lymphatic system that can cause lymph node obstruction. This cyst is <u>behind</u> the sternocleidomastoid muscle as opposed to the brachial cleft cyst, which is in front of the sternocleidomastoid muscle. Can be associated with Turner syndrome.

Hx/PE: Dysphagia, SOB, disfiguring, large mass on lateral neck.

Diagnosis:

- TSH and FT4 levels (to rule out thyroid dysfunction).
- Neck radiography, ultrasound, and MRI.

Treatment: Surgical excision.

Pediatric enuresis

Primary enuresis

Patients have not had a prolonged period of nighttime dryness.

Secondary enuresis

Involuntary nighttime urination while asleep, where the patient has had previous nighttime dryness and then reverts to bedwetting. Secondary enuresis can be associated with stressors in the patient's life such as divorce, conflicts, or a newborn sibling. Can be associated with family history.

Diagnosis:

- No work-up required if occurs <u>before</u> the age of 5 years and child is <u>a</u>symptomatic.

- If >5 years of age <u>or</u> symptomatic, need to rule out other causes of enuresis such as UTIs (urinalysis and urine culture), diabetes (fasting glucose), or diabetes insipidus (urine osmolality, serum osmolality, and urine sodium).
  - *Optimal initial test*: urinalysis (if positive result, than order urine culture).
  - If recurrent UTIs, perform VCUG.

Treatment:

- *Best initial therapy* is a non-pharmacologic approach (behavioral modifications), attempt for at least 3 months including fluid management, voiding before bedtime, positive encouragement, and eliminating late-evening fluid intake (at least 2 hours before bedtime).

- If above measures fail, **enuresis alarm** is a more active intervention and is the first line intervention.
  - If no improvement after enuresis alarm after 3 months than try pharmacologic approach.

- If non-pharmacologic approach fails, pharmacologic agents such as desmopressin (*first line treatment*) or imipramine (*second line treatment*) can be used for short-term treatment.

Pediatric development

Milestones

➢ 2 months: lifts head to 45 degrees and eyes follow to midline. Rooting reflex. Social smile.

➢ 4 months: lifts head to 90 degrees. Eyes can cross the midline. Recognizes people.

➢ 6 months: rolls over, grasps a rattle, feeds self, and knows parent from non-parent.

➢ 12 month: sits with support, pull themselves up to stand, and shows stranger anxiety. No Babinski reflex.

➢ 15 months: walks and says 1 or 2 words.

- 18 months: makes a tower of two blocks, says three words, and can use spoon and a cup.

- 2 years: can make a tower of 6 blocks, says 2-word sentences, runs and walks up the stairs. Parallel play.

- 3 years: can draw circles and say 3-word sentences, and has imaginary friends.

- 4 years: can draw squares and crosses, says 4-word sentences, dresses with assistance, and asks many questions.

- 5 years: draws stick figures and triangles, skips, and dresses and undresses without assistance.

Pediatric vaccinations

Vaccinations

- Egg-based vaccinations: IM influenza (is contraindicated in children with egg allergies [controversial]) and MMR (not contraindicated in children with egg allergies).

- Live vaccinations: MMR, influenza (nasal), rotavirus, varicella, yellow fever, and oral polio (Sabin).

- Pregnancy precautions: no MMR vaccination 1 month prior to pregnancy or during pregnancy (but not clinically backed up).

- HIV patients: cannot give BCG vaccination to HIV patients but can give MMR vaccination.

- IM Influenza vaccinations: cannot give to children younger than 6 months of age.

- Nasal Influenza vaccinations: cannot give to children younger than 2 years of age.

- *H. influenzae* type b vaccination (Hib): can be given at the age of 2 months, 4 months, 6 months, and 12 months.

- Meningitis vaccinations: usually given at age 11-12 years of age and a booster at age 16.

- DTaP × 5: given at 2 months, 4 months, 6 months, 15 months, and 4-6 years.

Fun facts:

✓ There is no need to decrease the vaccination dose or delay vaccination because of low birth weight or prematurity (give vaccinations at the chronological age).

✓ A person with mild to moderate fever can be vaccinated.

✓ Parents can legally refuse vaccinations, but this needs to be documented in the patient's chart.

✓ The MMR vaccination does not cause autism.

Childhood injury prevention

Preventative measures

➤ No solid foods until the age of 6 months.

➤ No cow milk until the age of >12 months.

➤ No honey until the age of >12 months.

➤ Child should sit in car seat backwards if aged <1 year or weighing <20 Ibs.

Pediatrics Index

A

acute hepatic encephalopathy 56
air contrast enema 28
amblyopia 54
annular pancreas 26
APGAR score 1
aplastic crisis 42
ataxia-telangiectasia 35
ATM protein 35
atrial septal defect 12

B

B12 deficiency 52
balloon atrial septostomy 14
bile acids 4
biliary atresia 3
bilirubin 3
brachial cleft cyst 58
bronchiolitis 37
Bruton's agammaglobulinemia 32
bubble baby disease 35

C

C1 esterase deficiency 36
C1 inhibitor concentrate 36
calcium deficiency 52
caput succedaneum 8
cardiac catheterization 11
cerebral palsy 47
Chediak-Higashi syndrome 36
choanal atresia 23
chronic granulomatous disease 34
clavicular fracture 8
clotrimazole cream 11
coarctation of aorta 13
common variable immunodeficiency 33
congenital diaphragmatic hernia 24
congenital umbilical hernias 30
conjunctivitis 5
constipation 31

crib death 54
cross eye 54
croup 38
cystic fibrosis 22
cystic hygroma 59

D

dacryostenosis 56
development 60
diaper candidiasis 10
diaper dermatitis 10
diarrhea 32
DiGeorge syndrome 34
diverticulectomy 29
diverting colostomy 24
Down syndrome 17
duodenal atresia 26
duodenostomy 27

E

Edwards syndrome 18
enuresis 59
epiglottitis 39
Erb-Duchenne palsy 8
erythema infectiosum 42
erythema toxicum 9
erythroblastosis fetalis 4
Ewing's sarcoma 50
exchange transfusion 4

F

febrile seizures 44, 47
fifth disease 42
folic acid deficiency 52
fragile X syndrome 22
Friedreich's ataxia 53

G

gastroesophageal reflux 31
gastroschisis 25

Index, cont'd

H

hand-foot-mouth disease 46
Henoch-Schonlein purpura 54
hepatitis B vaccination 5
Hirschsprung's disease 29

I

IgA deficiency 33
injury prevention 62
intussusception 27
iron deficiency 52
ivacaftor 22

J

jaundice 3

K

karyotype 20
Kasai procedure 4
Kawasaki disease 46
kernicterus 3
Klinefelter syndrome 20
Klumpke's palsy 8
Koplik's spots 42

L

Ladd's procedure 28
laryngotracheobronchitis 38
lazy eye 54
lead poisoning 57
lecithin-sphingomyelin ratio 2
leukemia 48
leukocoria 55
leukocyte adhesion deficiency 35
lymphocyte count 34
lysosomal trafficking regulator
protein 36

M

malrotation 28

management at delivery 2
McCune-Albright syndrome 21
measles 43
Meckel's diverticulum 29
Meckel's scintigraphy 29
meconium ileus 22
meningitis 40
milestones 60
Mongolian spots 10
mumps 43

N

nasal polyps 58
nasolacrimal duct probing 56
necrotizing enterocolitis 30
neuroblastoma 49
nitroblue tetrazolium test 34
N-myc 48
normal vital signs 1
NP-swab culture 37

O

obesity 32
omphalitis 35
omphalocele 25
osteosarcoma 50
ostium defect 12

P

parvovirus B19 42
Patau syndrome 19
patent ductus arteriosus 12
pertussis 39
phenobarbital-enhanced hepatobiliary scintigraphy 3
phenylketonuria 21
phototherapy 4
physiological jaundice 4
Prader-Willi syndrome 53
pyloric stenosis 26
pyloromyotomy 26
preventative measures 62

Index, cont'd

R

racemic epinephrine 38
rapid strep test 37
reflexes 7
renovascular disease 17
respiratory distress syndrome 2
retinoblastoma 55
retropharyngeal abscess 39
Reye's syndrome 47, 56
ribavirin 38
rickets 51, 53
rifampin 41
roseola 44
rubella 43

S

sarcoma botryoides 51
screening 6
severe combined immunodeficiency 35
shingles 45
shoulder dystocia 9
silo formation 25
skull fractures 7
slapped cheek 42
strabismus 55
subacute sclerosing panencephalitis 43
subconjunctival hemorrhage 7
sudden infant death syndrome 54
sweat chloride test 22
systolic murmurs 17

T

terminal complement deficiency 36
tetralogy of Fallot 15, 21
third heart sounds 17
throat culture 38
thymic shadow 57
thyroglossal duct cyst 58
total anomalous pulmonary venous
return 15
total complement activity 36
tracheal esophageal fistula 23
transient tachypnea of newborn 2
transposition of the great arteries 14
tricuspid atresia 16
truncus arteriosus 16
Turner syndrome 20

U

urinary tract infection 41

V

vaccinations 61
varicella 44
ventricular septal defect 11
vesicoureteral reflux 41
vital signs 1
vitamin D 5, 53
vitamin deficiencies 52
vitamin K 4
voiding cystourethrogram 41
volvulus 27
Von Hippel-Lindau syndrome 51

W

WAGR 49
whooping cough 39
Wilms' tumor 49
Wiskott-Aldrich syndrome 33

Z

zoster 45

www.ingramcontent.com/pod-product-compliance
Lightning Source LLC
Chambersburg PA
CBHW040837180526
45159CB00001B/214